WALL PILATES WORKOUTS FOR WOMEN OVER 50

7 Easy Steps by step Guide for seniors to lose weight, Achieve Mobility, Strength and good Balance With less Effort

Rachel J. Bradberry

TABLE OF CONTENT

INTRODUCTION

A woman named Stella lived in a little village surrounded by undulating hills and babbling brooks. Stella was known for her sweet demeanor and welcoming smile, yet beyond her outer appearance lay a deep battle.

Her days were filled with aches and pains, a continuous reminder of her sedentary lifestyle and lack of physical activity.
Stella's mornings started with a stiff awakening, her joints protesting each movement as she got out of bed.

The overall soreness that pervaded her body seemed to drag her down, putting a pall over her formerly bright spirit. Fatigue clung to her like a thick fog, clouding her thoughts and depleting her vitality before the day even began.

As the sun rose higher in the sky, Stella attempted to carry out her daily activities, but each step was greeted with opposition from her complaining joints. Simple tasks such as walking or bending were difficult, leaving her feeling discouraged and dissatisfied.

Despite her difficulties, Stella was determined to find a solution. She consulted specialists and tried numerous cures, but nothing appeared to bring long-term comfort. It wasn't until one fateful day, while wandering through a health bookstore, that Stella came across a faded this book

Stella, gently flicked over its pages, her eyes expanding with each discovery. Within its bindings was a treasure mine of wisdom, hidden mysteries hidden beneath the yellowed parchment. As she went further into its pages, Stella felt a spark of hope light within her tired heart.

Stella set off on a transformational adventure, armed with her newly acquired wisdom. She began adopting the book's principles into her everyday routine, such as gentle exercises and mindful activities. With each passing day, she felt the grip of anguish ease, being replaced with a renewed sense of vigor and power.

Stella's body gradually began to respond to the modest interventions of exercise and self-care. Her joints' rigidity began to melt away, giving way to a newfound suppleness that allowed her to move gracefully and effortlessly.
 The overall discomfort that had previously plagued her days faded away, replaced with a sensation of well-being that penetrated every fiber of her existence.

Stella reflected on her path and understood that the genuine secret to health and wellness had always been within her reach.

It was discovered not in transitory solutions or fast cures, but in the soft embrace of self-love and care. So, armed with the hidden secrets hidden behind the pages of a forgotten book, Stella regained her vigor and embraced a life of health, happiness, and limitless possibilities.

Chapter 1: Understanding Pilates Principles

Pilates is a popular kind of exercise that aims to strengthen the body, improve flexibility, and increase general fitness.

Pilates' guiding principles are crucial to the discipline, serving as the foundation for both successful and safe training. Understanding these concepts is essential for anyone wishing to begin a Pilates journey.

Pilates focuses on a certain style of breathing called "lateral thoracic breathing."

This entails breathing deeply through the nose, stretching the ribcage laterally, and exhaling thoroughly through the mouth, which activates the core muscles. Proper breathing makes activity easier, increases attention, and promotes calm.

Concentration: Pilates is more than just going through the movements; it demands mental attention and concentration on each action.

By remaining present and focused, practitioners may optimize the benefits of each practice while maintaining optimal posture and muscle engagement.

Pilates is really about control. The movements should be precise, purposeful, and graceful. Practitioners learn to control their bodies via a variety of exercises, progressively strengthening their strength, stability, and coordination.

Pilates centers on the notion of the "powerhouse," which includes the muscles of the belly, lower back, hips, and buttocks. Strengthening this region creates a firm foundation for movement and helps to prevent injury.

All motions start from the core, which promotes efficient and balanced muscular growth.

Precision: In Pilates, quality is prized above quantity. Each action should be executed with accuracy, with emphasis on appropriate alignment and muscle activation. This attention to detail not only improves outcomes but also reduces the chance of damage.

Flow: Pilates exercises are intended to flow effortlessly from one to the next, resulting in a seamless transition between movements. A Pilates workout relies heavily on fluidity and rhythm, which promote relaxation, circulation, and overall well-being.

Pilates seeks to integrate the mind and body by encouraging a stronger link between physical movement and mental awareness. Practicing breath, movement, and focus can help practitioners develop a harmonic balance of strength, flexibility, and control.

Individuals may get the full advantages of Pilates by learning and practicing these concepts, which range from improved posture and muscular tone to increased general health and well-being. Pilates, whether performed on a mat or with specialized equipment, provides a comprehensive approach to training that promotes longevity and vitality.

Benefits of Wall Pilates for Women Over 50

Wall Pilates is a modified version of classic Pilates that uses a wall to provide support and resistance, making it an excellent training choice for women over 50.

This mild yet effective workout provides several advantages targeted to the demands of this audience.

Improved Posture: As we age, maintaining appropriate posture becomes increasingly vital for avoiding back discomfort and preserving spinal health. Wall Pilates promotes spinal alignment and improves the core muscles that maintain healthy posture.

Increased Flexibility: As we age, our flexibility gradually declines, resulting in stiffness and a reduced range of motion. Wall Pilates combines stretching movements that target key muscle groups, hence improving flexibility and joint mobility.

Enhanced Strength: As we age, muscle mass tends to shrink, resulting in weakness and reduced functioning.

Wall Pilates uses the resistance supplied by the wall to build muscles throughout the body, particularly the core, arms, and legs, increasing total strength and balance.

Low-impact workouts are vital for maintaining joint health, particularly for people who have arthritis or other joint disorders.

Wall Pilates involves moderate motions that activate the joints without putting too much strain on them, enhancing joint health and lowering the chance of injury.

Balance and Coordination: As you become older, maintaining your balance and coordination becomes more difficult, increasing your chance of falling and being injured.

Wall Pilates combines balance and coordination exercises, which assist women over 50 improve their stability and lower their chance of falling.

Stress Relief: Exercise is considered to be a natural stress reliever, and Wall Pilates is no different. Wall Pilates incorporates concentrated movements and mindful breathing methods to help decrease stress and promote relaxation and well-being.

Improved Bone Density: Women over the age of 50 are more likely to develop osteoporosis, a disorder defined by reduced bone density.

Weight-bearing exercises, such as Wall Pilates, can help increase bone density and lower the risk of fractures.

Wall Pilates has various advantages for women over 50, including better posture, flexibility, strength, joint health, balance, coordination, stress alleviation, and bone density.

Women who incorporate this simple but effective workout into their regimen can improve their general health and well-being as they age.

Safety Tips and Precautions

As women get older, maintaining an active lifestyle becomes more crucial for their general health and well-being.

Wall Pilates is an excellent low-impact workout with multiple advantages, including increased strength, flexibility, and posture.

To guarantee a safe and successful workout, ladies over 50 must follow particular safety advice and measures when doing wall Pilates.

Consultation with a healthcare physician: Before beginning any new fitness plan, particularly if you are over 50, you should check with your healthcare physician.

They may analyze your general health and make tailored suggestions to ensure that wall Pilates is right for you.

Warm-Up and Cool-Down: Before commencing wall Pilates exercises, warm up your muscles and joints properly. Similarly, include a cool-down period to assist your body return to a resting condition and avoid post-exercise pain.

perfect Alignment and Form: Keep perfect alignment and form during each wall Pilates exercise. This involves maintaining a neutral spine, relaxed shoulders, and using your core muscles to support your back.

Start Slowly and Progress progressively: If you're new to wall Pilates or returning after a break, begin with simple exercises and progressively increase the intensity and complexity over time. Listen to your body and avoid pushing too hard, especially in the early phases.

Use Supportive Equipment: To improve your exercise safety and comfort, invest in high-quality supportive equipment such a

Pilates mat and robust wall-mounted Pilates machines.

Stay Hydrated and Take Breaks: Hydration is essential for any training regimen, so drink water before, during, and after your wall Pilates workout. Additionally, pay attention to your body's signals and take rests as required to avoid weariness and overexertion.

Avoid Overstretching: While flexibility is crucial, don't overstretch or force your body into awkward positions. Instead, concentrate on soft, controlled motions that build flexibility over time.

Chapter 2: Basic Wall Pilates Exercise

Pilates, a type of exercise that focuses on strengthening core muscles, increasing flexibility, and encouraging total body alignment, is especially useful for women over 50. As we get older, maintaining strength and flexibility becomes increasingly crucial for mobility and overall health.

Wall pilates exercises provide a safe and effective approach for women of this age to engage in low-impact workouts that focus on major muscle areas.

Below are some simple wall pilates exercises created exclusively for women over 50 to improve strength, flexibility, and posture.

1. *Wall Squats:*

Stand with your back to a wall and your feet hip width apart.

Slowly lower your body into a squat posture, maintaining your back against the wall and your knees in line with your ankles.

Hold the squat for 10-15 seconds before gently returning to the starting position.

Repeat for 10-15 repetitions, keeping perfect form and working your core muscles.

2. *Wall Planks:*

Stand facing the wall and place your hands on it, a little wider than shoulder width apart.

Walk your feet back until your body is in a straight line from head to heels, arms outstretched.

Hold this plank posture for 20-30 seconds, with your core engaged and your back straight.

To get back to where you started, move your feet carefully back towards the wall.

Repeat 3-5 times, progressively increasing the duration of the plank as you gain strength.

3. Wall push-ups:

Stand facing the wall, with your hands slightly wider than shoulder width apart and at shoulder height.

Walk your feet back so that your body forms a diagonal line from head to heels, arms outstretched.

Lower your chest towards the wall while maintaining your elbows close to your body.

Push yourself back up to the starting position, focusing on your chest and arm muscles.

Repeat for 10-15 repetitions, altering the effort by changing your body's angle to the wall.

4. Wall Bridges:

Lie on your back, feet flat on the wall, knees bent at a 90-degree angle.

Press your feet against the wall and elevate your hips to the sky, activating your glutes and core.

Hold the bridge posture for 10-15 seconds before slowly lowering your hips back to the floor.

Repeat for 10-15 repetitions, keeping a straight line from shoulders to knees throughout the action.

5. Wall Angels:

Stand with your back to the wall, feet hip width apart, and arms at your sides.

Slowly lift your arms upwards while maintaining them in touch with the wall, forming a "y" shape.

Lower your arms back to your sides, keeping contact with the wall during the action.

Repeat for 10-15 reps while maintaining your shoulders relaxed and your core engaged.

Incorporating these simple wall pilates exercises into a daily workout regimen will help women over 50 improve their strength, flexibility, and posture, resulting in better overall health and wellness.

Always get advice from a healthcare expert before beginning any new fitness regimen, especially if you have any pre-existing medical ailments or concerns.

Wall Squats and Lunges

In terms of lower-body empowerment, two exercises stand out as unexpected but formidable allies: wall squats and lunges. These exercises break convention, challenging traditional views of strength training with their novel approach to working many muscle groups at once.

Wall squats:

Imagine resisting gravity by leaning on a sturdy castle while your thighs engage in a silent war for strength. This is the essence of the wall squat.

As you lower yourself into a squat, your quadriceps, hamstrings, and glutes awaken, creating a power symphony.

Your core functions as a conductor, maintaining proper alignment and stability. With each breath, you descend deeper into the pit of power, retaining your place like a warrior defending their country.

Lunges:

Step into the world of lunges, where balance and coordination are paramount.

Each thoughtful step involves your entire lower body in a dance of control and accuracy.

Your quadriceps, hamstrings, and glutes coordinate their efforts, driving you forward with purpose.

As you lower yourself into the lunge, your core acts as an anchor, keeping you stable amid the frenzy of movement.

With each repetition, you shape not just your muscles but also your thoughts, establishing a link between power and elegance.

Unveiling Unseen Benefits:

Beyond the physical realm, wall squats and lunges provide an opportunity for self-discovery and empowerment.

They challenge your preconceived views of strength, encouraging you to embrace the uncommon and find beauty in the fight.

Through endurance and dedication, you can discover secret stores of strength inside yourself, overcoming the boundaries of the everyday.

Embrace the unusual. Embrace the task. Accept the power of wall squats and lunges as you go on a path of self-discovery and empowerment.

With each repetition, you reinvent what it means to be strong, tough, and unmistakably distinctive.

Wall Push-Ups and Chest Press

Wall push-ups and chest press workouts are two great ways to build upper-body strength. Both target the chest, shoulders, and triceps muscles, although they differ in terms of equipment and muscle engagement.

In this tutorial, we'll go over the specifics of each exercise, such as appropriate technique, benefits, and variants.

Wall push-ups.

Form: Stand at arm's length facing a wall, with your hands slightly wider than shoulder-width apart. Maintain a straight body from head to heels.

Bend your elbows to lower your chest towards the wall, then push yourself back to the starting position.

Wall push-ups are a beginner-friendly exercise that helps to increase upper body strength and endurance.

They also promote shoulder stability and are an excellent choice for people who have sustained wrist or shoulder problems.

To make the push-ups more challenging, position your feet farther away from the wall or execute them on an inclined surface. For less intensity, stand closer to the wall or do knee push-ups.

Chest Press

Form: recline on a flat bench with one dumbbell in each hand, palms facing away from you. Extend your arms up until the dumbbells are directly over your shoulders. Lower the dumbbells to your chest in a controlled way, then raise them back to their starting position.

Benefits: Chest press workouts work the pectorals, shoulders, and triceps. They assist in increasing upper-body strength, muscular mass, and symmetry. Chest presses also train stabilizing muscles in the core and build functional strength.

The chest press may be performed with a variety of equipment, including barbells, resistance bands, and machines. In addition, incline or decline bench angles may be modified to target specific parts of the chest.

Including wall push-ups and chest press movements in your training program can result in considerable gains in upper-body strength, muscular tone, and general fitness.

Whether you're a novice or an experienced lifter, these workouts provide a variety of alternatives for meeting your fitness objectives.

Wall Plank Variation

Wall plank variants are useful workouts for women over 50 to strengthen their core muscles, improve stability, and increase overall fitness. These exercises are low-impact, making them appropriate for people who have joint problems or mobility limits that come with age. Here is a complete guide to executing wall plank variations:

1. Wall Planks:

Begin by standing facing a wall about an arm's length away.

At shoulder height, place your hands on the wall and lean forward

Walk your feet back until your body is in a straight line from head to heels.

Hold this position for 20–30 seconds, keeping your core muscles engaged and your breathing steady.
Repeat for 2-3 sets, progressively increasing the time as you gain strength and endurance.

2. Wall Plank With Leg Lift:

Begin in the wall plank posture, hands on the wall, body aligned.

Lift one leg off the ground while maintaining it straight and parallel to the floor.

Before lowering the leg back down, hold for a few seconds

Switch to the other leg and repeat.

Aim for 8-10 repetitions on each leg for 2-3 sets, concentrating on stability throughout.

3. Wall Plank With Arm Reach:

Assume the wall plank stance, keeping your body steady and aligned.

Lift one arm off the wall and extend it forward, parallel to the ground.

Hold for a few seconds, then return to your starting position.

Repeat with the opposing arm.

Perform 8-10 repetitions of each arm for 2-3 sets, focusing on balance and control.

Benefits:

Strengthens core muscles such as the abdominals, obliques, and lower back, which are essential for posture and spinal stability.

Enhances stability and balance, lowering the danger of falls and accidents.

Improves general body awareness and proprioception, which are essential for effective motion in everyday life.

Can be readily tailored to individual fitness levels and develop over time.

Including wall plank variants in a daily workout regimen can help women over 50 keep a strong, stable core and enhance overall fitness, resulting in a healthier, more active lifestyle.

Always consult a healthcare expert before beginning any new workout regimen, especially if you have pre-existing health ailments or concerns.

Chapter 3: Intermediate Wall Pilates Routines

Pilates is an excellent kind of exercise for women over 50, providing several advantages such as increased strength, flexibility, and posture.

Intermediate wall Pilates exercises are a tough yet safe approach to maximizing these advantages while working on core stability and balance. This is a detailed introduction to intermediate wall Pilates exercises designed exclusively for ladies over 50.

1. Wall Roll-Downs: Begin by standing with your back against the wall and your feet hip-width apart. Inhale to stretch your spine, then exhale as you slowly roll down one vertebra at a time, pressing your lower back against the wall. Hold for a second before inhaling and rolling back up. Repeat 8 to 10 times.

2. *Wall Squats:* Stand back against the wall, feet hip-width apart. Slide down the wall into a squat position, keeping your knees behind your feet. Hold for a few breaths before pushing through your heels to return to standing. Repeat 10 to 12 times.

3. *Wall Planks:* To begin, place your hands shoulder-width apart on the wall and take a step back, forming a straight line from head to heels. Engage your core and hold for 30-60 seconds, keeping your hips aligned with your shoulders.

4. *Wall Bridge:* Lie on your back, feet against the wall, knees bent. Press your feet against the wall and elevate your hips to the ceiling, using your glutes and hamstrings.

Before Slowly lowering back down, hold for a few breaths

Repeat 8 to 10 times.

5. *Wall Leg Circles:* Lie on your back, one leg stretched against the wall, the other towards the ceiling. Circulate the extended leg in both directions while maintaining your core engaged and hips steady. Repeat 5–8 repetitions, then switch legs.

6. *Wall Chest Opener:* Stand facing the wall, one hand at shoulder height. Rotate your body away from the wall while maintaining your arm straight to feel a stretch in your chest and shoulders.

Before switching sides, hold for at least 30 seconds

Incorporating these intermediate Wall Pilates exercises into your fitness program will help women over 50 increase their strength, flexibility, and general well-being while also fostering better posture and balance. Always remember to listen to your body and alter activities to meet your specific requirements and abilities.

Side Leg Lifts and Leg Circles

Side leg lifts and leg circles are two powerful exercises that target lower-body muscles, namely the hips, thighs, and glutes. Incorporating these movements into your training program will help increase lower-body strength, stability, and flexibility while exercising the core muscles.

Side leg lifts:

To begin side leg lifts, lie on your side with your legs straight and stacked on top of each other. Place your head on your lower arm and your upper hand on the floor in front of you for support. Engage your core muscles to keep your body stable during the workout.

Next, elevate your upper leg as high as possible without twisting your hips or tilting your body. Keep your leg straight and don't bend your knee. Hold the raised posture for a second before slowly lowering your leg back to the starting position. Repeat the exercise for the required amount of times, then switch to the opposite side.

Leg Circles:

Leg circles begin by lying on your side, but this time bend your lower leg slightly for increased stability. Keep your upper leg straight and lift it slightly off the ground. Point your toes and use your core muscles.

Begin by forming little circles with your upper leg, starting from the hip joint. Concentrate on regulating the movement and remaining stable throughout.

Gradually raise the size of the circles while maintaining control and precision. After you have completed the rings in one direction, flip to the opposing direction. Repeat the appropriate amount of times, then move to the opposite side.

Benefits:

Both movements work the muscles of the outer thighs, hips, and glutes, improving strength, stability, and tone in these regions. They also exercise the core muscles, resulting in improved posture and stability.

Furthermore, these workouts can assist increase hip and thigh flexibility, which can enhance general mobility and function.

Include side leg lifts and leg circles in your training program to improve lower-body strength and stability while also exercising the core muscles.

Wall Bridge and Hip Lifts

Wall bridges and hip lifts are great workouts for developing your core, lower back, glutes, and hamstrings. They engage many muscle areas at once, making them effective complements to any training plan. Here is a complete breakdown of these exercises:

Wall bridges:

Setup: Lie on your back with your feet flat on the ground and your knees bent at a 90° angle. Place your arms at your sides for stability.

Execution: Engage your core and push your lower back into the floor. Lift your hips off the ground so that your body forms a straight line from shoulders to knees.

Hold for a second before lowering back down with control.

Wall bridges generally work the glutes, hamstrings, and lower back muscles. They also activate the core to maintain stability.

Variations: To add difficulty, try single-leg wall bridges by extending one leg straight and elevating the hips. You may also increase the difficulty by adding a weight or resistance band across your hips.

Hip Lifts:

Setup: Begin in a similar posture as wall bridges, lying on your back with your feet flat on the ground and your knees bent. Arms can be at your sides or extended for balance.

Lift your hips off the ground by tightening your glutes and pressing through your heels. Concentrate on forming a straight line from shoulders to knees. Hold at the peak for a bit before lowering back down with control.

Hip lifts focus largely on the glutes, hamstrings, and lower back. They also use the core muscles to maintain stability and balance.

Variations: To boost intensity, attempt single-leg hip lifts, which include extending one leg straight and elevating the hips. You may also increase the difficulty by adding a weight or resistance band across your hips.

Incorporating wall bridges and hip lifts into your training program will help you gain core and lower body strength, stability, and endurance. Start with excellent form and progressively increase intensity for the best results.

Wall Teaser and Roll-Downs

When it comes to morning workouts, women want programs that are efficient, effective, and flexible to their hectic schedules. Incorporating wall teasers and roll-downs into your morning regimen may provide a full-body exercise that targets many muscle groups while increasing flexibility and core strength.

Wall teasers are a diverse workout that focuses on the upper body, including shoulders, arms, and core muscles. To do wall teasers, face a wall with your feet hip-width apart and arms outstretched at shoulder height, palms placed on the wall.

Lower your body slowly toward the wall, bending your elbows while maintaining your core engaged and your spine neutral. When your face is near to the wall, push yourself back up to the beginning position using your chest and arm muscles. Repeat for a certain number of times, concentrating on controlled motions and appropriate technique.

Roll-downs are an effective exercise for developing spine mobility, hamstring flexibility, and core strength. Start by standing tall, with your feet hip-width apart and your arms at your sides.

Slowly articulate your spine as you roll down to the floor, beginning with your chin tucked into your breast and gradually lowering each vertebra until your hands reach the floor or as far as you feel comfortable.

Pause in this forward fold position and feel the stretch in your hamstrings and back. Engage your core and steadily roll back up to standing, stacking each vertebra one at a time until you reach the beginning position. Repeat for a certain number of times, concentrating on smooth, controlled motions and breathing.

Incorporating wall teasers and roll-downs into a morning workout regimen provides women with a complete approach to fitness, addressing many muscle groups while encouraging flexibility, mobility, and core strength.

These workouts are readily customized to meet individual fitness levels and goals, making them appropriate for both beginners and expert exercisers. Women can benefit from these workouts by following them consistently and with appropriate technique.

Chapter 4: Advanced Wall Pilates Techniques

Advanced Wall Pilates Techniques transform basic Pilates exercises by using the wall as a multifunctional instrument for added support, resistance, and refinement.

These approaches exemplify the blend of innovation and tradition, enhancing the advantages of Pilates and cultivating a stronger mind-body connection.

Wall Squats: Start by placing your back firmly against the wall, feet hip-width apart, and arms stretched forward.
Slowly descend into a squat, keeping your back on the wall and your knees aligned with your ankles.

This precise technique engages the quadriceps, glutes, and core with unrivaled precision, promoting lower-body strength and stability while developing perfect form and alignment.

Standing facing the wall, form a solid foundation with feet hip-width apart and arms gracefully stretched aloft. As you glide down towards the wall, softly articulate each vertebra and allow your fingertips to skim its surface.

This beautiful yet demanding action lengthens the hamstrings and calves while reinforcing the core with unshakable control and delicacy, resulting in increased spinal mobility and overall postural integrity.

Wall Planks: Take a plank stance, feet against the wall and hands firmly placed beneath your shoulders.

Engage your core, glutes, and thighs while holding this powerful posture for a lengthy period of time, appreciating the exquisite challenge of maintaining perfect alignment despite the slight oscillations caused by the wall's presence. This dynamic variant creates a symphony of muscle engagement, shaping the core, shoulders, and arms while also developing a strong sense of balance and proprioception.

Wall Teasers: Lying supine with legs beautifully stretched against the wall and arms gracefully poised overhead, begin a harmonic climb to your toes, using the entire force of your core to orchestrate this gorgeous movement.

This beautiful blend of strength and elegance captures the essence of Pilates, improving mind-body synergy and shaping the core, hip flexors, and upper body with unmatched refinement and accuracy.

Wall Side Planks: Accept the challenge of lateral stability as you lie on your side, feet braced on the wall and forearm acting as a sturdy anchor. As you bask in the exhilaration of completing this hard achievement, raise your hips to the skies, forming a smooth line of alignment from head to heels.

This transcending workout strengthens the obliques, hips, and shoulders while cultivating a profound feeling of balance and poise in the face of ever-changing gravitational currents.

Accept the transformational power of these Advanced Wall Pilates Techniques, as they take your practice to new heights of strength, stability, and profound body awareness.

Wall Scissors and Bicycle Crunches

As women age, keeping a strong core becomes more crucial for their general health and mobility.

Wall scissors and bicycle crunches are two powerful exercises designed exclusively for ladies over 50 who want to improve their abdominal muscles while reducing impact on other parts of their body.

Wall Scissors:

Setup: Start by lying flat on your back, buttocks near a wall. Extend your legs up against the wall to establish a 90-degree angle with your torso. Place your hands flat on the ground at your sides to provide support.

Execution: Engage your core muscles and steadily lower one leg to the floor, holding the other leg against the wall. Alternate your legs in a scissor-like action, ensuring control and stability throughout the movement.

Repetitions: Aim for 2-3 sets of 10-15 repetitions each leg, increasing as your strength develops.

Benefits:

Targets the lower abdominal muscles without putting tension on the neck or back.
improves core stability and balance.
Adjusting the angle of the legs on the wall allows for easy adaptation to individual fitness levels.

Bike Crunches:

Setup: Lie on your back, knees bent, feet flat on the floor. Place your hands loosely behind your head, elbows pointed to the sides.

Execution: Raise your shoulders off the floor while using your core muscles. To replicate a biking action, bring your right elbow towards your left knee while straightening your right leg. Repeat on the opposite side, bringing your left elbow to your right knee.

Repetitions: Aim for 2-3 sets of 15-20 repetitions each side, with emphasis on controlled movements and perfect form.

Benefits:

Targets the upper and lower abdominal muscles, as well as the obliques.
Increases total core strength and endurance.

The speed and range of motion may be simply modified to meet the fitness needs of any individual.
Incorporating wall scissors and bicycle crunches into a daily training regimen can

assist women over 50 keep a strong and stable core, which benefits general health and functional mobility as they age. Always consult a healthcare expert before beginning any new workout regimen, especially if you have pre-existing health concerns.

Wall Roll-Ups and Teaser Variations

Women over 50 must maintain a strong and flexible physique for their general health and well-being. Pilates exercises such as wall roll-ups and teaser variants can help people improve their core strength, flexibility, and posture while also lowering their risk of injury.

These exercises target important muscular areas, such as the core, back, and thighs, and may be tailored to specific fitness levels.

Wall Roll-ups:

Set up: Stand with your back against a solid wall, feet hip-width apart, and arms stretched overhead.

Execution: Roll down your spine, one vertebra at a time, until your back is flat on the wall. As you roll back to the beginning position, engage your core muscles.

Variations: For novices, bend your knees slightly to relieve tension on the lower back.

As you improve, consider straightening your legs for a more difficult workout. You may further boost the intensity by wrapping a resistance band around your thighs.
Teaser Variations:

Traditional Teaser: Sit on a mat, legs out in front of you, feet flexed. Lean back slightly and raise your legs off the ground while balancing on your sit bones to engage your core.
Extend your arms forward and elevate your torso to create a V shape. Hold for a few breaths before carefully lowering back down.

Modified Teaser: Begin in the same posture as the regular teaser, but with your feet on the ground. Lift one leg at a time while staying balanced and using your core. This form puts less tension on the lower back while still addressing the core muscles.

Teaser with Twist: Perform the standard teaser, but when you elevate your torso, spin your upper body to one side and stretch your opposing hand toward the outside of the lifted leg.

Return to the middle, then repeat on the opposite side. This version provides an additional challenge by activating the obliques.

Women over 50 who incorporate wall roll-ups and teaser variants into their training program can increase their strength, flexibility, and posture, resulting in a healthier and more active lifestyle.

Always listen to your body and check with a fitness professional before beginning any new workout regimen.

Wall Plank with Knee Tucks and Pike

As women get older, maintaining core strength and stability becomes more vital for their general health and mobility.

The wall plank with knee tucks and pike is a fantastic exercise for strengthening the core, shoulders, and hip flexors while improving balance and posture. This detailed instruction will guide you through the right form and technique for carrying out this exercise safely and successfully.

Step 1: Getting in Position

Find a clear wall space. With arms length away, approximately stand facing the wall

Assume the plank position:

Place your hands flat on the wall, shoulder height and little wider than shoulder width apart. Step back until your body creates a straight line from head to heels, engaging your core and maintaining a neutral spine.

Step 2: Performing the Exercise

Knee Tucks: Hold the plank posture and slowly bring one knee towards your chest, using your abdominal muscles. Hold for a second, then restore your foot to its initial position. Repeat on the opposite side.

On each leg 10 to 12 repetitions should be aimed at.

Pike: From a plank posture, engage your core and raise your hips to the sky, producing an inverted V shape with your body.

Keep your legs straight and your heels pressed against the ground. Hold for a second before lowering back into plank position. Aim for 8–10 repetitions.

Step 3: Tips for Success

Focus on form: Maintain core engagement throughout the workout to preserve your lower back and increase efficacy.

Control your movements: To properly activate the muscles, perform each action gently and controllably.

Modify as required. If the complete plank posture is too difficult, begin by completing the knee tucks and pike against a higher surface, such as a solid table or countertop.

Incorporate the wall plank with knee tucks and pike into your normal exercise program to strengthen your core, enhance balance, and maintain your general mobility as you age.
Always contact a healthcare expert before beginning any new fitness regimen,

especially if you have any pre-existing medical ailments or concerns.

Chapter 5: Adding Props into Wall Pilates

Including props in wall Pilates for women over 50 can improve the efficacy of their training routines by offering extra support, stability, and resistance.

Wall Pilates provides various advantages to this group, including increased posture, core strength, flexibility, and balance. Women over 50 can enhance these advantages by using props such as resistance bands, stability balls, and foam rollers in their exercises to meet their unique needs.

Resistance bands are one of the most commonly utilized props in wall Pilates for women over 50. These bands have varying resistance levels and may be used to target particular muscle areas, including the arms, legs, and core.

For example, adding a resistance band across the thighs during wall squats can assist engage the glutes and thighs while also supporting the knees.

Stability balls are another useful tool for wall Pilates workouts. These inflatable balls provide an element of instability, which further activates the core muscles during workouts like wall squats, wall sits, and wall push-ups.

Stability balls may also be used for modest stretching and balancing exercises, which improve posture and reduce the chance of falling.

Foam rollers are a fantastic prop for women over 50 who do wall Pilates because they help relieve tension in tight muscles and promote flexibility. Incorporating foam rolling movements into a regular Pilates regimen can help reduce stiffness in the back, hips, and shoulders, improving general mobility and range of motion.

Props in wall Pilates for women over 50 can improve the efficacy of their exercises by offering extra support, stability, and resistance.

Resistance bands, stability balls, and foam rollers are just a few of the props that may be used to target particular muscle areas, increase flexibility, and encourage improved posture and balance.

Women over 50 may tailor their exercises to their specific requirements and goals by including these props into their regimens, resulting in a stronger, healthier, and more active lifestyle.

Using Resistance Bands for Added Challenge

LResistance bands are becoming increasingly popular among women over 50 who want to add variation and challenge to their fitness regimens.

These adaptable and portable pieces of equipment have several advantages, including increased strength, flexibility, and balance, making them an excellent alternative for women seeking to maintain or improve their fitness as they age.

One of the most significant benefits of employing resistance bands is their ability to deliver varying resistance over a range of motion. This means that when you stretch the band, the resistance rises, providing a more effective workout than traditional weights.

This is especially useful for women over 50 since it prevents muscle loss and maintains bone density, both of which are essential for general health and mobility.

Resistance bands also allow for a variety of exercises that target different muscle areas. Focusing on exercises that increase functional motions like squats, lunges, rows, and presses can assist women over 50 retain their independence and quality of life as they become older.

Resistance bands may be readily added to these workouts to provide an additional challenge and promote muscle activation.

Resistance bands are soft on the joints, making them a safer choice for ladies with arthritis or other joint disorders that come with age.

The regulated resistance produced by the bands enables smooth, fluid motions without putting unnecessary stress on the joints, lowering the risk of damage.

In addition to strength training, resistance bands may be used for flexibility and balance exercises, which are critical for preserving mobility and lowering the risk of falls as women age.

Stretching with resistance bands can assist increase flexibility and range of motion, whilst balance exercises can aid with stability and coordination.

Including tension bands in a workout regimen may provide various benefits to women over 50, including increased strength, flexibility, and balance, all of which are critical for preserving health and independence as they age.

Resistance bands are a wonderful tool for ladies who want to stay active and vibrant into their golden years because to their variety and ease of usage.

Incorporating Stability Balls for Core Engagement

Stability balls, often known as exercise balls or Swiss balls, are multipurpose instruments that can help increase core activation during exercises.

By including stability balls in your training program, you may increase the efficiency of standard core exercises while also increasing balance, coordination, and stability. Here's how.

Improved Core Activation: Stability balls provide an element of instability, forcing your core muscles to work harder to maintain balance and stability during training. This enhanced activation results in better muscle recruitment and a more efficient core workout.

Stability balls may be used to do a variety of workouts that target different parts of the core, such as the rectus abdominis, obliques, and transverse abdominals.

There are several workouts that test and improve your core, ranging from simple crunches and planks to more sophisticated movements such as stability ball rollouts and pikes.

Improved Balance and Coordination: Balancing on a stability ball activates not just your core muscles but also stabilizer muscles all around your body. This improves general balance and coordination, which are required for useful movements in everyday life and sports.

Versatility and accessibility: Stability balls are inexpensive, portable, and appropriate for all fitness levels. Whether you're a novice trying to improve your core strength or an experienced athlete looking to add a new challenge to your exercises, stability balls may be readily included into your regimen.

Stability ball activities strengthen deep core muscles, such as the transverse abdominis and multifidus, in contrast to standard core workouts, which predominantly target surface muscle groups. Strengthening these muscles is critical for maintaining spinal stability and preventing injuries.

Stability balls are extremely useful instruments for improving core engagement and general fitness. Integrating stability ball exercises into your program allows you to increase core activation, enhance balance and coordination, and target a wider variety of core muscles.

Whether you're working out at home, the gym, or even the workplace, stability balls are a simple and effective method to take your core training to the next level.

Utilizing Foam Rollers for Balance and Flexibility

Foam rolling is an excellent and accessible technique for women over 50 to improve their balance and flexibility. As we get older, maintaining these areas of physical fitness becomes more vital for overall health and injury prevention.

 Foam rollers, which are cylindrical pieces of foam, are often used for self-myofascial release, a type of self-massage that works on tight muscles and connective tissues.

To begin, choose a foam roller that is suitable for your needs. To strike the right mix between efficacy and comfort, choose a medium-density roller.

Begin with a warm-up to stimulate blood flow and prepare the muscles for foam rolling. This may involve modest cardiovascular activity or dynamic stretching.

When you're ready, carefully and methodically roll over the foam roller to target certain muscle areas. Concentrate on regions prone to tension and pain, such as the calves, quadriceps, hamstrings, glutes, and upper back.

Apply the required pressure with smooth motions and adjustments to your body posture. When you find a tender region, pause and breathe deeply to enable the muscle to relax and release tension.

Foam rolling not only helps muscles relax, but it also enhances proprioception, or the body's understanding of its location in space. This improved proprioception promotes greater balance and stability, lowering the likelihood of falls and accidents, which is especially relevant for women over the age of 50.

Furthermore, including foam rolling into your daily practice can help with flexibility by increasing joint range of motion. This is especially useful for preserving mobility in joints prone to stiffness, such the hips and shoulders.

Consistency is essential to reaping the full advantages of foam rolling. Include foam rolling activities in your weekly fitness routine, either after workouts or as part of a specific recuperation session.

 Begin with a few minutes of foam rolling for each muscle group, gradually increasing time and intensity as your body responds.

Foam rolling is an effective technique for ladies over 50 to enhance their balance and flexibility. With good technique and consistency, it can help relieve muscular tension, improve proprioception, and increase overall physical well-being. Incorporate foam rolling into your regimen to help you achieve your fitness goals and stay active as you age.

Chapter 6: Customizing Wall Pilates Workouts

Pilates, which emphasizes core strength, flexibility, and alignment, is an ideal kind of exercise for women over 50. Tailoring Pilates movements to use a wall as a support aid offers a level of stability and balance that is critical for this group.

Here's a complete guide on designing wall Pilates programs for ladies over 50:

Warm-up: Start with mild motions to warm up your body and stimulate blood flow. Neck rolls, shoulder shrugs, and ankle circles might help to loosen up stiff muscles.

Alignment Check: In Pilates, proper alignment is critical to preventing joint strain. Use the wall as a reference point for proper posture, ensuring that the head, shoulders, hips, and heels are aligned.

Wall Squats: Squat with your back against the wall to develop your quadriceps, glutes, and core muscles. This exercise increases lower-body strength and stability, which are necessary for daily tasks.

Wall Push-Ups: Face the wall at arm's length and execute push-ups against it. This variation puts less tension on the wrists and shoulders while still exercising the chest, shoulders, and triceps.

Wall Angels: Lie on the floor, back against the wall, knees bent, feet flat. Extend your arms upward while retaining touch with the wall, then gently drop them down to resemble angel wings. This workout focuses on shoulder mobility and stability.

Wall Bridge: Lie on the floor, feet against the wall and knees bent. Lift your hips off the floor, activating your glutes and hamstrings. This exercise strengthens the posterior chain and increases pelvic stability.

Wall Roll-Downs: Stand with your back against the wall and your feet hip-width apart. Roll slowly down the spine, articulating each vertebra before returning to the top position. This exercise increases spinal mobility and flexibility.

Cool down and stretch: After the workout, do some simple stretches to enhance flexibility and relieve muscular tension. Concentrate on stretches that target the hamstrings, hip flexors, and chest.

Customizing Pilates sessions with the assistance of a wall is a safe and effective technique for women over 50 to increase strength, flexibility, and balance, thereby improving their overall quality of life.

Adapting Exercises for Individual Needs and Limitations

Women's bodies change as they age, which might impact their capacity to participate in some sorts of exercise.

However, being active and leading a healthy lifestyle are critical for general well-being, particularly for women over 50. To guarantee a safe and efficient fitness plan, workouts must be modified to meet individual demands and limits.

1. Assessing Individual Needs: Before developing an exercise program, it is critical to determine each woman's particular requirements. Fitness level, medical history, existing health issues, and personal objectives are all important considerations.

Consulting with a healthcare expert or a trained fitness trainer can help you adapt a program to your specific needs.

2. Low-Impact Cardiovascular workouts: Low-impact cardiovascular workouts are great for women over 50 since they promote heart health and increase general endurance without placing too much strain on the joints.

Walking, swimming, cycling, and utilizing elliptical machines are all terrific exercise alternatives. These exercises' intensity and length can be changed to suit individual fitness levels and limits.

3. Strength Training: Strength training routines are essential for preserving muscle mass, bone density, and functional strength as women age. However, it is critical to select workouts that are suited for your specific demands and limits.

Bodyweight exercises, resistance band workouts, and mild weightlifting with appropriate form can all assist develop strength and flexibility while avoiding injury.

4. *Flexibility and Balance:* Stretching exercises are critical for preserving flexibility and avoiding injuries, particularly as women age. Gentle yoga or Pilates practices can assist increase flexibility, balance, and core strength. These workouts can be tailored to meet any physical limits or constraints.

5. *Listening to the Body:* As women get older, it's crucial to listen to their bodies and make the necessary changes to their workout regimens. Paying attention to any discomfort or pain during exercises and changing routines as needed is critical for avoiding injuries and achieving long-term fitness and wellness.

Adapting workouts for women over 50 necessitates a tailored strategy that takes into account their specific requirements and limits. Women may maintain their overall health and fitness by implementing a mix of low-impact aerobic, strength training, flexibility, and balancing activities.

Consulting with healthcare specialists and trained fitness trainers can help you build a safe and successful workout program based on your specific needs.

Designing Personalized Wall Pilates Routines

Designing Personalized Walls Pilates routines for women over 50 require a careful approach that meets their specific requirements and limitations while encouraging strength, flexibility, and general well-being.

Pilates, which emphasizes regulated movements and core strength, is an ideal type of exercise for women in this demographic since it may help improve posture, balance, and joint health.

When developing a tailored regimen, it is critical to consider the individual's fitness level, any preexisting health concerns, and specific goals.

Women over the age of 50 are more likely to experience concerns like decreasing bone density, arthritis, or lower back discomfort; thus workouts should be selected or changed accordingly.

Begin by thoroughly assessing the client's physical ability, including any areas of stiffness, weakness, or pain.

This evaluation will help guide the selection of activities and changes to ensure a safe and productive workout. Core strength exercises, such as pelvic tilts and leg slides, can assist increase stability and support for the spine.

Using the wall as a prop offers diversity to the routine by supporting balance and alignment while raising the intensity of some routines.

For example, wall squats can help to strengthen the lower body and improve functional movement patterns. Wall push-ups can also help to strengthen the upper body while avoiding wrist strain.

Flexibility is another important factor to consider, as maintaining or enhancing range of motion can assist prevent injuries and improve general mobility. Stretching exercises like wall angels and chest openers can help relieve tension in the shoulders and chest while also improving posture.

Throughout the routine, emphasize correct breathing methods and mindful movement, urging the client to focus on the link between their breath and movement in order to relax and reduce tension.

As with any training regimen, progression is essential. As the client gains strength and familiarity with the exercises, changes can be made to increase the difficulty and stimulate further growth in strength, flexibility, and general fitness.

Regular review and consultation with the client will ensure that the routine is suited to their specific requirements and goals, promoting long-term adherence and success.

Modifying Intensity Levels for Progression or Recovery

As women age above 50, their fitness requirements change, necessitating careful consideration of effort levels for both advancement and recuperation.

Whether you're looking to improve your fitness or recover from an injury, controlling your intensity correctly is critical for getting the best results and overall health.

1. Progress:

Women over 50 can advance in fitness by progressively increasing the intensity of activities to challenge the body and encourage strength and endurance increases. Here's how to change intensity levels effectively:

Begin slowly by doing low to moderate-intensity workouts like walking, swimming, or easy yoga to provide the groundwork.

Gradual raise: Gradually raise intensity by adding resistance, increasing pace, or introducing intervals to test the muscles and cardiovascular system without overworking them.

Listen to the body: Pay heed to indications from your body. If you're feeling tired or uncomfortable, reduce your activity to avoid overexertion and injury.

Functional Training: Use functional workouts that mirror everyday motions to enhance balance, stability, and general functionality.

2. Recovery:

As women age, recovery becomes increasingly crucial in terms of injury prevention, fatigue management, and overall well-being. Here's how to adjust intensity levels for optimal recovery:

Active healing: Engage in low-intensity exercises like walking, cycling, or mild stretching to enhance blood flow and muscle healing while reducing stress.

Mind-Body Practices: Use mind-body techniques such as meditation, tai chi, or mild yoga to reduce stress, enhance sleep quality, and promote general relaxation and healing.

Proper Nutrition and Hydration: To assist healing processes, eat nutrient-dense meals and remain hydrated throughout the day.

Prioritize excellent sleep to allow the body to heal and revitalize, with a goal of 7-9 hours of undisturbed sleep every night.

Women over 50 may improve their fitness journey while lowering their risk of injury and increasing general health and well-being by adjusting intensity levels correctly for progression and recuperation. To attain long-term fitness objectives, you must listen to your body, advance slowly, and emphasize recuperation.

Chapter 7: Maintaining Consistency and Progress

Maintaining consistency and growth for women over 50 is critical to their overall health and lifespan.

Women entering this period of life frequently encounter specific obstacles relating to health, employment, and personal fulfillment.

By focusing on consistency and development, women may overcome these obstacles and attain their objectives more successfully.

Physical Health: Women over 50 must be consistent in their efforts to maintain a healthy lifestyle.

Regular exercise, a healthy diet, and enough sleep are all necessary components.

At this age, strength training is more necessary for maintaining muscle mass and bone density. Progress may be monitored by gradually increasing endurance, flexibility, and general physical fitness.

Mental Well-Being: Consistently practicing mindfulness, meditation, or relaxation techniques can help manage stress and improve mental clarity.

Continued study, hobbies, and social ties can all help you improve your mental health. Reading, solving puzzles, and learning new skills can all help improve cognitive health.

Career and Personal Development: Women over 50 may confront obstacles in their employment, such as age discrimination or managing transformations.

Consistency in skill development, networking, and exploring chances for improvement is key. Advancements in one's job, following new hobbies, or meeting personal objectives are all ways to assess progress.

Health Screenings and Preventive Care: It is critical to schedule regular health checkups and screenings for disorders such as breast cancer, osteoporosis, and heart disease. Progress in preventative care requires being proactive in addressing any health risks and implementing appropriate lifestyle changes.

Financial Stability: Consistency in financial planning and budgeting is essential for women over 50, particularly as they approach retirement. Smart investments, savings techniques, and obtaining expert assistance when needed can all help you make progress.

Embracing Change: Being consistent in adapting to life changes, such as empty nesting or retirement, is critical. Progress entails seizing new possibilities, exploring new pathways, and achieving contentment at this stage of life.

Women over 50 may enjoy meaningful, healthy, and purposeful lives by being consistent in crucial aspects of their lives and pushing for development. It is critical to prioritize self-care, create attainable objectives, and celebrate progress along the way.

Setting Realistic Goals and Tracking Progress

Setting realistic goals and evaluating progress is critical for women over 50 to stay motivated, healthy, and achieve their objectives. As women age, their bodies and lives change, making it even more vital to create attainable objectives based on their unique requirements and skills.

1. Assess Current Health and Fitness Levels: Before making any goals, women over 50 should evaluate their current health and fitness levels. This may entail meeting with healthcare providers, undergoing a thorough physical checkup, and recognizing any restrictions or health issues that may impact goal planning.

2. Define Clear and precise objectives: Women over 50 should set clear and precise objectives that are both attainable and appropriate to their age, lifestyle, and fitness level. Setting realistic objectives, whether they be for cardiovascular health, muscle strength, or weight management, can help you stay focused and motivated.

3. Divide Large Goals into Smaller, More Manageable Steps: Dividing bigger goals into smaller, more manageable steps can help them feel less daunting and measure progress more easily. For example, if the aim is to lose weight, breaking it down into monthly or weekly goals helps make the process more manageable.

4. Incorporate range and Balance: Women over 50 should include a range of exercises and activities in their fitness program to avoid boredom, lower the chance of injury, and enhance overall fitness. This might involve a combination of aerobic, strength, flexibility, and balancing exercises.

5. *Track Progress on a Regular Basis:* Tracking progress is critical for remaining accountable and motivated. Women over 50 can utilize a variety of strategies to measure their progress, including maintaining a workout log, utilizing fitness tracking apps, and scheduling frequent check-ins with a fitness coach or trainer.

6. *alter Goals as Needed:* As women over 50 move through their fitness journey, it's critical to frequently examine and alter their goals as necessary.

This might include adjusting the intensity or frequency of workouts, making new objectives to push oneself, or addressing any difficulties or failures that may happen.

Setting realistic objectives and evaluating progress is critical for women over 50 to maintain good health, fitness, and general well-being. Women over 50 may stay inspired and empowered on their fitness path by reviewing their present circumstances, setting clear objectives, breaking them down into achievable stages, introducing diversity and balance, tracking progress on a regular basis, and revising goals as needed.

Overcoming Plateaus and Challenges

As women go through life, they face numerous hurdles and plateaus, particularly as they approach the age of 50 and beyond. This population frequently encounters unique challenges that demand perseverance, effort, and a planned strategy to overcome.

Here's a detailed guide to help women over 50 manage and conquer these plateaus and challenges:

Health and wellness: As women age, physical health becomes more vital. Overcoming plateaus in fitness and wellbeing necessitates a personalized approach that combines regular activity, balanced nutrition, and relaxation.

Consulting with healthcare specialists can assist in developing individualized programs to address particular health challenges while maintaining general well-being.

Career Advancement: Many women over 50 may feel stuck in their jobs or encounter age-based discrimination in the workplace.

Overcoming this plateau entails staying current with industry trends, learning new skills through training programs or education, networking with people from all generations, and using their experience and knowledge to pursue leadership positions or entrepreneurial enterprises.

Financial Security: Women over the age of 50 may find it difficult to plan for retirement and maintain financial security.

Overcoming financial plateaus entails budgeting, investing intelligently, getting financial counsel, investigating new income sources such as freelancing or consulting, and taking proactive efforts to guarantee their financial future.

Personal Growth and Development: Overcoming plateaus in personal growth necessitates self-reflection, creating new goals, pushing beyond one's comfort zone, accepting change, and maintaining a positive attitude.

Hobbies, lifelong learning, and seeking mentorship or peer support may all help with ongoing personal growth.

Maintaining meaningful social ties becomes increasingly important for women over 50, particularly when children leave the nest and social networks shift.

To battle feelings of isolation and loneliness, overcome social plateaus by actively participating in community activities, joining clubs or groups with similar interests, attending social events, and cultivating connections.

Embracing Aging: Society frequently fosters negative misconceptions about aging, which can lower women's self-esteem and confidence.

Overcoming this plateau entails accepting aging as a normal part of life, concentrating on inner strengths and knowledge gained over time, exercising self-care, and being surrounded by supportive people who appreciate aging gracefully.

Women over 50 may overcome plateaus and problems by focusing on four important areas and adopting a proactive mentality, allowing them to live fulfilled lives with confidence and perseverance.

Incorporating Variety and Fun into Wall Pilates Workouts

Incorporating variation and enjoyment into wall Pilates exercises for women over 50 is not only possible but also necessary for sustaining interest and getting the full advantages of the training program.

By incorporating creativity and diversity into their routines, women in this demographic may improve their strength, flexibility, and general well-being while having fun.

To begin, using the wall provides a new dimension to conventional Pilates movements, providing extra support and stability while pushing the core muscles.

Begin with basic exercises like wall squats and leg lifts, then proceed to more difficult motions like wall push-ups and aided inversions. This variety not only works different muscle areas but also gives individuals a sense of success as they overcome new hurdles.

Props like resistance bands, tiny balls, and foam rollers can help to improve the training experience.

These instruments provide resistance, help, or instability, increasing the efficacy of workouts and keeping the program interesting.

For example, using a resistance band into leg lifts or arm exercises increases training intensity while maintaining joint integrity and functional strength.

Including mindfulness and relaxation practices into your routine can improve the mind-body connection and reduce stress. Adding breathing exercises, meditation, or moderate stretches against the wall can help women over 50 relax and unwind while reaping the physical advantages of Pilates.

Including social contact into wall Pilates sessions can improve their enjoyment and sustainability. Group courses or virtual sessions allow women to interact, share stories, and inspire one another, cultivating a feeling of community and accountability.

Incorporating diversity and pleasure into wall Pilates routines for women over 50 is both possible and helpful.

Women in this demographic may improve their physical and mental well-being while enjoying the road to improved health and vitality by trying new workouts, using props, increasing mindfulness, and encouraging social engagement.

CONCLUSION

Firstilall Pilates provides low-impact, high-intensity workouts tailored to the specific needs of women over 50.

Wall Pilates, with its emphasis on controlled movements and alignment, provides a safe setting for building strength, flexibility, and balance, all of which are important components in preserving mobility and preventing common aging-related problems.

The versatility of wall Pilates exercises allows for customized workouts based on individual fitness levels and health problems.

Whether you're a novice or a seasoned practitioner, the adaptability of wall Pilates routines offers a gradual and sustainable approach to exercise for women over 50, encouraging long-term commitment and success.

Furthermore, the use of the wall as a prop adds a new dimension to basic Pilates movements, providing greater stability and support.

This feature is especially useful for women over 50, who may struggle to maintain balance and stability owing to age-related problems or past accidents.

Wall Pilates uses the wall as a tool for resistance and alignment, allowing participants to use muscles more efficiently while putting less strain on joints and ligaments.

The attentive aspect of wall Pilates promotes a deeper connection between the body and mind, resulting in relaxation and stress reduction. As women over 50 deal with life transitions and obligations, the contemplative components of wall Pilates provide a comprehensive approach to wellbeing, improving mental clarity and emotional resilience.

Wall Pilates emerges as a comprehensive workout solution tailored specifically to women over 50, meeting their individual demands and goals.

Wall Pilates teaches women how to accept aging with grace and energy by combining components of strength, flexibility, balance, and mindfulness, encouraging a lifetime path of health and well-being.

Wall Pilates, as a diverse and accessible workout modality, can help promote active aging and improve the overall quality of life for women over 50.

THANK YOU PAGE

Thank you for selecting this book. Your support is really appreciated. Similarly, I am grateful for the purchase of this book.

Your input is valuable; please share your ideas in a review. It serves as a reference for future improvements. Enjoy reading and utilizing it!

Workout exercise planner to Track and check Progress

Workout Planner for seniors

	EXERCISE	GOAL
MON DAY		
TUES DAY		
WEDNES DAY		
THURS DAY		
FRI DAY		
SAT DAY		

Workout Planner for seniors

	EXERCISE	GOAL
MON DAY		
TUES DAY		
WEDNES DAY		
THURS DAY		
FRI DAY		
SAT DAY		

Workout Planner for seniors

	EXERCISE	GOAL
MON DAY		
TUES DAY		
WEDNES DAY		
THURS DAY		
FRI DAY		
SAT DAY		

Workout Planner for seniors

	EXERCISE	GOAL
MON DAY		
TUES DAY		
WEDNES DAY		
THURS DAY		
FRI DAY		
SAT DAY		

Workout Planner for seniors

	EXERCISE	GOAL
MON DAY		
TUES DAY		
WEDNES DAY		
THURS DAY		
FRI DAY		
SAT DAY		

Workout Planner for seniors

	EXERCISE	GOAL
MONDAY		
TUESDAY		
WEDNESDAY		
THURSDAY		
FRIDAY		
SATDAY		

Workout Planner for seniors

	EXERCISE	GOAL
MON DAY		
TUES DAY		
WEDNES DAY		
THURS DAY		
FRI DAY		
SAT DAY		

Workout Planner for seniors

	EXERCISE	GOAL
MON DAY		
TUES DAY		
WEDNES DAY		
THURS DAY		
FRI DAY		
SAT DAY		

Workout Planner for seniors

	EXERCISE	GOAL
MON DAY		
TUES DAY		
WEDNES DAY		
THURS DAY		
FRI DAY		
SAT DAY		

Workout Planner for seniors

	EXERCISE	GOAL
MON DAY		
TUES DAY		
WEDNES DAY		
THURS DAY		
FRI DAY		
SAT DAY		

Workout Planner for seniors

	EXERCISE	GOAL
MON DAY		
TUES DAY		
WEDNES DAY		
THURS DAY		
FRI DAY		
SAT DAY		

Workout Planner for seniors

	EXERCISE	GOAL
MONDAY		
TUESDAY		
WEDNESDAY		
THURSDAY		
FRIDAY		
SATDAY		

Workout Planner for seniors

	EXERCISE	GOAL
MON DAY		
TUES DAY		
WEDNES DAY		
THURS DAY		
FRI DAY		
SAT DAY		

Workout Planner for seniors

	EXERCISE	GOAL
MON DAY		
TUES DAY		
WEDNES DAY		
THURS DAY		
FRI DAY		
SAT DAY		

Workout Planner for seniors

	EXERCISE	GOAL
MON DAY		
TUES DAY		
WEDNES DAY		
THURS DAY		
FRI DAY		
SAT DAY		

Workout Planner for seniors

	EXERCISE	GOAL
MON DAY		
TUES DAY		
WEDNES DAY		
THURS DAY		
FRI DAY		
SAT DAY		

Workout Planner for seniors

	EXERCISE	GOAL
MON DAY		
TUES DAY		
WEDNES DAY		
THURS DAY		
FRI DAY		
SAT DAY		

Workout Planner for seniors

	EXERCISE	GOAL
MONDAY		
TUESDAY		
WEDNESDAY		
THURSDAY		
FRIDAY		
SATDAY		

Workout Planner for seniors

	EXERCISE	GOAL
MON DAY		
TUES DAY		
WEDNES DAY		
THURS DAY		
FRI DAY		
SAT DAY		

Workout Planner for seniors

	EXERCISE	GOAL
MON DAY		
TUES DAY		
WEDNES DAY		
THURS DAY		
FRI DAY		
SAT DAY		

Workout Planner for seniors

	EXERCISE	GOAL
MON DAY		
TUES DAY		
WEDNES DAY		
THURS DAY		
FRI DAY		
SAT DAY		

Workout Planner for seniors

	EXERCISE	GOAL
MONDAY		
TUESDAY		
WEDNESDAY		
THURSDAY		
FRIDAY		
SATDAY		

Workout Planner for seniors

	EXERCISE	GOAL
MON DAY		
TUES DAY		
WEDNES DAY		
THURS DAY		
FRI DAY		
SAT DAY		

Workout Planner for seniors

	EXERCISE	GOAL
MONDAY		
TUESDAY		
WEDNESDAY		
THURSDAY		
FRIDAY		
SATURDAY		

Workout Planner for seniors

	EXERCISE	GOAL
MON DAY		
TUES DAY		
WEDNES DAY		
THURS DAY		
FRI DAY		
SAT DAY		

Workout Planner for seniors

	EXERCISE	GOAL
MON DAY		
TUES DAY		
WEDNES DAY		
THURS DAY		
FRI DAY		
SAT DAY		

Workout Planner for seniors

	EXERCISE	GOAL
MON DAY		
TUES DAY		
WEDNES DAY		
THURS DAY		
FRI DAY		
SAT DAY		

Workout Planner for seniors

	EXERCISE	GOAL
MON DAY		
TUES DAY		
WEDNES DAY		
THURS DAY		
FRI DAY		
SAT DAY		

Workout Planner for seniors

	EXERCISE	GOAL
MONDAY		
TUESDAY		
WEDNESDAY		
THURSDAY		
FRIDAY		
SATDAY		

Workout Planner for seniors

	EXERCISE	GOAL
MON DAY		
TUES DAY		
WEDNES DAY		
THURS DAY		
FRI DAY		
SAT DAY		

Workout Planner for seniors

	EXERCISE	GOAL
MON DAY		
TUES DAY		
WEDNES DAY		
THURS DAY		
FRI DAY		
SAT DAY		

Workout Planner for seniors

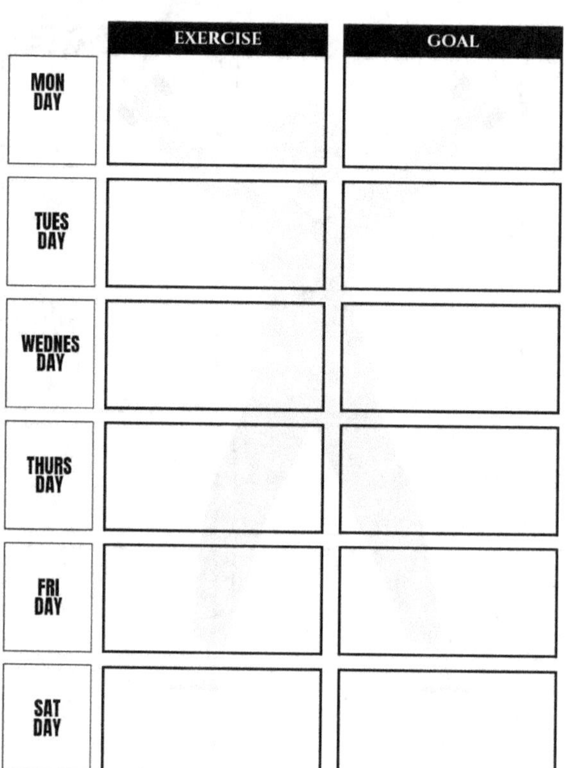

Workout Planner for seniors

	EXERCISE	GOAL
MON DAY		
TUES DAY		
WEDNES DAY		
THURS DAY		
FRI DAY		
SAT DAY		

Workout Planner for seniors

	EXERCISE	GOAL
MON DAY		
TUES DAY		
WEDNES DAY		
THURS DAY		
FRI DAY		
SAT DAY		

Workout Planner for seniors

	EXERCISE	GOAL
MON DAY		
TUES DAY		
WEDNES DAY		
THURS DAY		
FRI DAY		
SAT DAY		

Workout Planner for seniors

	EXERCISE	GOAL
MON DAY		
TUES DAY		
WEDNES DAY		
THURS DAY		
FRI DAY		
SAT DAY		

Workout Planner for seniors

	EXERCISE	GOAL
MON DAY		
TUES DAY		
WEDNES DAY		
THURS DAY		
FRI DAY		
SAT DAY		

Workout Planner for seniors

	EXERCISE	GOAL
MON DAY		
TUES DAY		
WEDNES DAY		
THURS DAY		
FRI DAY		
SAT DAY		

Workout Planner for seniors

	EXERCISE	GOAL
MON DAY		
TUES DAY		
WEDNES DAY		
THURS DAY		
FRI DAY		
SAT DAY		

Workout Planner for seniors

	EXERCISE	GOAL
MON DAY		
TUES DAY		
WEDNES DAY		
THURS DAY		
FRI DAY		
SAT DAY		

Workout Planner for seniors

	EXERCISE	GOAL
MON DAY		
TUES DAY		
WEDNES DAY		
THURS DAY		
FRI DAY		
SAT DAY		

Workout Planner for seniors

	EXERCISE	GOAL
MON DAY		
TUES DAY		
WEDNES DAY		
THURS DAY		
FRI DAY		
SAT DAY		

Workout Planner for seniors

	EXERCISE	GOAL
MON DAY		
TUES DAY		
WEDNES DAY		
THURS DAY		
FRI DAY		
SAT DAY		

Workout Planner for seniors

	EXERCISE	GOAL
MON DAY		
TUES DAY		
WEDNES DAY		
THURS DAY		
FRI DAY		
SAT DAY		

Workout Planner for seniors

	EXERCISE	GOAL
MON DAY		
TUES DAY		
WEDNES DAY		
THURS DAY		
FRI DAY		
SAT DAY		

Workout Planner for seniors

	EXERCISE	GOAL
MON DAY		
TUES DAY		
WEDNES DAY		
THURS DAY		
FRI DAY		
SAT DAY		

Workout Planner for seniors

	EXERCISE	GOAL
MON DAY		
TUES DAY		
WEDNES DAY		
THURS DAY		
FRI DAY		
SAT DAY		

Workout Planner for seniors

	EXERCISE	GOAL
MON DAY		
TUES DAY		
WEDNES DAY		
THURS DAY		
FRI DAY		
SAT DAY		

Workout Planner for seniors

	EXERCISE	GOAL
MON DAY		
TUES DAY		
WEDNES DAY		
THURS DAY		
FRI DAY		
SAT DAY		

Workout Planner for seniors

	EXERCISE	GOAL
MON DAY		
TUES DAY		
WEDNES DAY		
THURS DAY		
FRI DAY		
SAT DAY		

Workout Planner for seniors

	EXERCISE	GOAL
MON DAY		
TUES DAY		
WEDNES DAY		
THURS DAY		
FRI DAY		
SAT DAY		

Workout Planner for seniors

	EXERCISE	GOAL
MON DAY		
TUES DAY		
WEDNES DAY		
THURS DAY		
FRI DAY		
SAT DAY		

Workout Planner for seniors

	EXERCISE	**GOAL**
MON DAY		
TUES DAY		
WEDNES DAY		
THURS DAY		
FRI DAY		
SAT DAY		

Workout Planner for seniors

	EXERCISE	GOAL
MON DAY		
TUES DAY		
WEDNES DAY		
THURS DAY		
FRI DAY		
SAT DAY		

Workout Planner for seniors

	EXERCISE	GOAL
MON DAY		
TUES DAY		
WEDNES DAY		
THURS DAY		
FRI DAY		
SAT DAY		

Workout Planner for seniors

	EXERCISE	GOAL
MON DAY		
TUES DAY		
WEDNES DAY		
THURS DAY		
FRI DAY		
SAT DAY		

Workout Planner for seniors

	EXERCISE	GOAL
MON DAY		
TUES DAY		
WEDNES DAY		
THURS DAY		
FRI DAY		
SAT DAY		

Workout Planner for seniors

	EXERCISE	GOAL
MON DAY		
TUES DAY		
WEDNES DAY		
THURS DAY		
FRI DAY		
SAT DAY		

Workout Planner for seniors

	EXERCISE	GOAL
MONDAY		
TUESDAY		
WEDNESDAY		
THURSDAY		
FRIDAY		
SATDAY		

Workout Planner for seniors

	EXERCISE	GOAL
MON DAY		
TUES DAY		
WEDNES DAY		
THURS DAY		
FRI DAY		
SAT DAY